Sexy Prostate

Male G-Spot Massage
For Pleasure and Health

For all men
and the women who love them

Erika Thost MD

Published by Erika Thost MD
SexyProstate.com

Produced by Wayne Marshall,
kaizen-marketing.com

Copyright © Erika Thost MD 2016
All rights reserved

Acknowledgements

I would like to acknowledge and appreciate the people from whom I learned so much, even though they may not know me personally:

Pamela Madison
Joseph Kramer PhD
David Wise PhD and Rodney Anderson MD
Jack Morin PhD
Jeanette Potts MD
Charlie Glickman PhD
Susie Bright
Carol Queen PhD and Robert Lawrence DC, EdD
Charles Muir
Barbara Carrellas
Dr Patti Taylor
Steven Braveman LMFT
Human Awareness Institute
Body Electric School
Nicole Daedone, One Taste
Jaiya

Praise for Sexy Prostate

"This is a much needed and timely resource for couples' sexual enhancement. The stigma of 'prostate massage' can take a back door, now that this information has been presented so well by Dr. Erika in this new guide."|
— Dr. Patti Britton, Clinical Sexologist, Co-Founder of SexCoachU.com, and host of over 40 couples' sexual enhancement DVDs

"I found this book very engaging and accessible. If sex education and counseling, in general, could be addressed in such a natural and pragmatic way, I believe this world would be a better place and sex therapy would be rarely required. Dr Erika's book satisfies a curiosity which frequently arises in clinical consultations. I will recommend her book to all the patients who (timidly) inquire about prostate sexual stimulation or to any couples asking to expand their repertoire and nurture or enhance their intimacy."
—Jeannette Potts MD, Men's Health Specialist. Editor / author of urological textbooks: *Essential Urology, Genitourinary Pain and Inflammation,* and *Men's Health.*

"Dr. Thost takes the prostate out of the Dr.'s office and into the bedroom. She demystifies prostate health and pleasure in her playful and easily accessible style."
—Jacqueline Richard, Psy.D., AASECT Certified Sex Therapist

"Loved it! Dr. Thost's book, Sexy Prostate, is very well-written, educational and fun with specific information for both men and women on how to navigate a long overlooked arena in human sexuality — the pleasuring of the prostate. A definite breakthrough for heightening the sexual experience. A must read!"
— *A.R.C., LMFT*

"An approachable tone to a sensitive topic"
—*Linda Leviton, LMFT. Author of Peace Within, Peace Between: Your Relationship Toolkit.*

"Dr Erika knows how important the prostate is, and what's more, she knows how much pleasure it can give. Easy for any partner to learn, her instructions are key to prostate health and bliss."
— *Carol Queen, co-author of The Sex & Pleasure Book: Good Vibrations Guide to Great Sex for Everyone. Director, The Center for Sex & Culture, San Francisco*

"Dr. Thost has compiled important information that can change lives in so many positive ways. This book is entertaining, fun, and opens up new vistas of health pleasure. I highly endorse it."
—*Thomas A. Reaper, MD, MPH*

Disclaimer

This information is for information and entertainment purposes only. It is not intended to be a substitute for medical diagnosing nor treatment nor medical advice. Please do not consider anything in this book or website as medical advice.

While this information is as accurate as possible, there are no guarantees or warranties for the complete accuracy of this information. Please always check with your doctor before you rely on any of this information for yourself.

Every man should have a urologist and an internist and have his prostate health checked by them on a regular basis. Please consult your physician promptly if there are any questions about the suitability of any of this information for you and if you have any medical questions.

More information about this topic is in the chapter on safety.

Table of Contents

Welcome to Prostate Massage 1
The Benefits of Prostate Massage 5
Prostate Pleasure Primer 11
Worried about Messy? 15
Genital Massage 27
External Prostate Massage 27
External Anal Massage 37
Getting Inside 43
Internal Anal Massage 49
Prostate Massage 53
Prostate Milking 61
Putting It All Together 63
Love Those Quickies! 69
Safety First 75
Supplies 79
Positions 85
Sex Toys 89
Therapeutic Prostatic Massage 97
Epilogue 101

Welcome to Prostate Massage

Welcome to the no-embarrassment guide to prostate massage. If you are a woman, you will learn how to massage your partner's prostate for both pleasure and health and how to find great satisfaction in the role. If you're a man, you will discover how prostate stimulation can make your orgasms both stronger and more profound. You'll also discover how to achieve a very different kind of orgasm, a unique addition to male sexual pleasure.

Here, you'll find out that the prostate is not just a mysterious appendage that is dormant until it begins to cause health problems late in life. It is actually an active sex organ, ready and willing to add new dimensions to your sex life.

For a woman, it can be fun to "do" your guy; to be in charge and give him lots of pleasure. What's more, it is easy for you to do him: easy, as in "not hard work" and easy as in "not hard to learn." And did I mention that the prostate or male G-spot is easy to find?

You may notice that this book is oriented towards straight couples. Of course, it can also work well for gay couples. However, in my experience, it is the straight men and the heterosexual couples who most need encouragement and information for exploring prostate pleasure. And there are few resources for them. So it is my mission to expand straight couples' sexual repertoire, and improve prostate health in the process!

Many straight men - well, most, once they give it a try - love prostate stimulation. For a woman, it can be a huge thrill to have your finger on his prostate during his orgasm, a chance to share his pleasure as in no other way. And for the man, you haven't lived if you haven't had her finger on your prostate during orgasm.

Here is a miracle that almost no one knows about, not even most doctors: during orgasm the prostate puffs out and gets bigger and firmer, and then contracts back to normal.

This book will make you curious about exploring the prostate. It will also get you ready to relax and let the good things happen. To get the most out of this book, I suggest you read the whole thing, then go back and review the topics that grab your attention.

In the early chapters, you'll find the practical information to start your prostate exploration, including how to prevent messiness. In the chapters following, the steps for prostate massage are clearly explained: how to get inside, how to avoid causing pain, how to touch the prostate itself.

Then we'll put it all together: what a session of male G-spot play looks like from beginning to end. And last, I'll throw in a few tips on how both of you can get the very most from the experience.

ERIKA THOST MD

The Benefits of Prostate Massage

Some people wonder: since it all seems like a hassle, with opportunities galore for misunderstanding and embarrassment, why bother?

Most men, after all, have not been anticipating the experience all their lives. They haven't missed what they haven't ever known. And they don't yearn for the chance to discover the male G-spot. So, why do it?

First and most important, this massage can make your orgasm deeper and somehow more complete. As one man in my workshop put it, "My orgasm is more draining, in a really good way." Actually he's right, literally as well as figuratively: orgasm accompanied by prostate massage can produce a greater volume of ejaculate and more intense contractions, prolonging the experience and making it more ecstatic.

The potential for these deeper experiences may build with recurring prostatic massage. So there is incentive to hang in there. Some men feel prostate pleasure right away. For others, it can take a little time and practice to get there.

Usually we assume that the male orgasm includes an ejaculation, and in this book I will assume that, too. However, men can have orgasms without ejaculation. Male G-spot massage is one way to learn about that other kind of orgasm. With a non-ejaculatory orgasm, you feel sensations in the whole body centering on the prostate. It is just a different - and, by all accounts, a pretty remarkable - sort of pleasure.

Don't worry, these other orgasms will not ruin the ones you already know and love. Indeed, they will not change them or diminish them. You get to have a unique pleasure in addition to the pleasure that you have now. The yummy sensations from the prostate are a learned and new kind of sensation.

Perhaps not surprisingly, the learning experience parallels that of woman's with the G-spot. Her G-spot may not feel good to her at first. Later as the sensations become more familiar, they become fun and orgasmic. And like women's experience with the G-spot, the feelings for the man can be more "interesting" in nature, with more nuance than the explosive joy of a "regular" orgasm. The prostate produces a very different type of sensation than the penis, one with greater subtlety and a more enduring emotional experience.

However, to access that learned pleasure fully, one has to start and end with a penis made happy by genital massage. This way, the new prostate sensations are anchored to something that is a tried-and-true source of fun.

Do confess: you probably took my allusion to the health benefits of prostate massage with a grain of salt, a harmless crutch to get more timid readers past the guilt and/or embarrassment. In fact, there is pretty solid evidence supporting the cod liver oil aspect of prostatic massage.

Yes, it really is good for you. It can relieve the symptoms of chronic prostatitis and the less well understood sources of chronic pelvic pain. It can also reduce prostate enlargement, which causes problems with peeing and sexual function. At this point there is not much research on whether massage helps to prevent these conditions from developing. But I have spoken with many urologists who, based on their patients' experience, have become advocates.

While we're at it, let's dispose of another myth. Contrary to what you may have been taught, there is a great deal of research that shows sex is good for your health. Just in case you need a little encouragement, several studies have shown that frequent enough ejaculations are associated with a lower risk of prostate cancer. And the payoff may be even bigger: many studies show a correlation between more frequent sex and longer life.

Let me introduce another virtue of prostate massage: it gives men a chance to experience the pleasure of playing a more passive role in sex. Men usually have the more active role for all sorts of reasons. They work hard physically during sexual intercourse, and their sexuality is totally visible since that erect penis is not exactly subtle. So it is a different experience for guys to just receive, to give up being in charge for a while, to explore the part of their sexuality that is hidden and vulnerable.

With prostatic massage the man also gets to learn about the pleasures of the anus, and there sure is a lot of potential for pleasure there. That can be a new and surprising experience for him.

Another advantage of male prostate pleasure is that no erection is needed. So it works well when there is not much erection happening for whatever reason. And, with the help of a toy (really a device), a man can do prostate massage for himself, by himself, an experience analogous to masturbation and its underrated pleasures.

ERIKA THOST MD

Prostate Pleasure Primer

We are not going to talk about prostate problems or cancer in this book. There are many resources for that available elsewhere. Our focus is purely on having fun with this mysterious organ.

First some basics. You pronounce the word "prostate" not "prostrate". There is just one 'r'. The first part is "pro", as in "I'm pro-prostate". The second part is "state" as in "state of arousal".

So how are the prostate and the male G-spot different? They aren't. The prostate is the anatomical name of the gland, and the male G-spot is a name for the functional area that produces the sensations. But I use them interchangeably.

Sometimes guys say, "My orgasms are just fine. I don't want to take the chance of having them changed." I want to reassure you that you'll still have orgasms just like the ones you have now. We just want to add to what you already get, not take anything away.

When you learn about sexuality, you need to listen with your heart and guts as well as with your brain. As you do new things, keep checking in with yourself. See if the information makes sense, if it feels good in your heart, and see if your gut feeling is positive.

I will present information that comes from my brain. I'm also trying to put into words the emotions that come up during erotic and intimate exploration. But I am using words to explain things that are inherently non-verbal. So some of it may not make a lot of sense to you, or at least not right away. Take your time and see if your emotions and your gut feelings can comprehend what the brain might not quite understand.

In a similar vein, my teaching about the prostate involves not just the nuts and bolts, but how to explore on your own. How you and your partner can do something totally new together: something that may not be immediately comfortable, that may require talking to each other in a different way, and that may make one or both of you feel vulnerable.

I'm not just going to tell you about the prostate, but also about the process of sexual and emotional exploration with your partner. Take what you want and leave the rest, make it your experience. There is no right or wrong way to use this book. Use it in a way that works for both of you.

The term "sexy prostate" sounds like an oxymoron, doesn't it? The prostate is not sexy, never has been and never will be. That's what we usually think, right? Well, you'll soon be thinking differently. The G-spot can give the guy pleasure, and its exploration can give both of you a greater sense of intimacy.

People have all kinds of feelings about the prostate. Men are (cautiously) curious about it because they have one. And they don't really know much more than the fact that it causes problems in middle age and brief embarrassment at their annual physicals. For women, the prostate is this mysterious thing that no one ever talks about.

I did a series of interviews with men about the subject. They saw the prostate as inscrutable and somewhat yucky when they were young, as in "Please, do we really need to talk about that?" And nothing but trouble when older. Clearly, we have a public relations problem here. My mission is to revitalize this poor maligned gland's image.

Actually, the prostate doesn't just sit there, it is active and, with sex, exciting. It does this cool thing, ballooning before ejaculation. It goes poof, rapidly growing bigger and firmer. Once in a class someone asked me, "Does it really make that poof noise?" My answer was, "It depends on how sensitive your ears are."

In any case, the expansion is so dramatic that it does not really need sound effects. So for the gal, you get some fascinating information there. When the prostate puffs out, the guy feels, "I'm gonna come now." If you, the woman, have your finger on his G-spot, you will notice that 'poof' and you'll know what it means. And you'll say to yourself, "Oh!" And a second later, you'll hear him say, "Oh!" Isn't it fun to have (literally) inside information like that about when he's going to come?

Even when I was in medical school, even when I was formally studying sexuality, no one ever mentioned this thing about the prostate. Hard to believe, isn't it? There you see: the prostate has way more going for it than we give it credit for.

Worried about Messy?

Lots of people worry about how to deal with the potentially messy part of butt play. But the reality is a lot tamer than one might imagine. It's easy!

First, and foremost: the issue of safety and cleanliness. There are definitely microorganisms in the butt area, but they are not the sort of pathogens that scientists dress up in space suits to avoid. So it is nice to be clean, but there's no need to be antiseptic. A quick clean up with a handy wipe all that is truly needed.

If you prefer, take a shower or a brief hot tub soak before. Maybe you'll do that together, as part of your foreplay. I do not recommend a long leisurely shower, bath or jacuzzi before playing, however. It tends to make people sleepy and slow. So save it for afterwards.

Do use soap, but not a lot because that can irritate the sensitive skin down there. Also, limit the vigor of your scrub for the same reason.

If either or both of you prefer less hair on the butt - this is about personal taste, not hygiene - it is easy to shave there with a regular safety razor. Afterwards, use a cream like benzoyl peroxide (over the counter, at the drug store) to prevent itching.

Yes, folks are hesitant to approach the butt because they worry about the messy part. They feel, reasonably enough, that the butt is supposed to be a one-way road. And it is an exit to stuff that we've been taught from toddlerhood to consider disgusting. But concern about the yuck factor is by far the biggest. As a wiseass cracked at one of my workshops, "What's everyone's number 1 worry? - Number 2."

And then, of course, everyone is concerned about the opposite issue - things going into their butt. Will it hurt? Will it make me gay? And what would mom think (shudder)?

Answering those question in no particular order... No, it will not hurt. It will not even be uncomfortable if you do it carefully, the way I describe in a later chapter. Actually it should feel good.

Will it make me gay? No, that is not how sexual orientation works. You're just enjoying a pleasurable part of your body. What would mom think? Well, I don't know. But even she was young once. Perhaps she'd say (or at least think) "Hey! Have some fun. I wish I'd tried that."

So let's put this in perspective. You've probably heard the line that no one on his death bed wishes that he or she had spent more time at the office. The fact is that people usually regret the things that they wanted to do but did not do, not the stuff they did do.

Now imagine yourself on your death bed, not anytime soon, of course. Would you rather be saying, "I was always really curious about exploring more sex stuff, like anal play, but the risk of messy was just too dreadful so I never did that." Or would you rather be gloating, "Well! We sure tried some crazy sex stuff. Some worked great and some flopped. But wow! Did we have fun!" Pretty clear choice, right?

For a really great experience, for some powerful and intense orgasms, for entering realms you didn't know existed, would you put up with the risk of a little messiness? Of course you would.

Now about the information provided in this book: nowhere else will you find it in such detail. People just do not talk about this topic at length. But I really want you to have the whole truth, so that you will realize it is not a big deal. Be prepared for some detailed discussion of your rectum and your anus (this is where the fourth graders in sex ed class giggle). Probably more detail than you've ever heard before. And yes, we will definitely be talking about poop (more giggles).

All doctors, by the way, have to get used to the subject pretty early on because they do hundreds of digital - which means finger - rectal exams (with gloves on). Then they even take any tiny bit of fecal matter from the glove and put it on a special paper to test for blood in the stool. Also, doctors routinely do procedures in the anal area. So as a physician, I long ago accepted that the area as just another body part.

Doctors try hard not to be embarrassed because it would be unprofessional, and because they understand it makes their patients more uncomfortable than necessary. Plus, doctors need to instruct people on how to collect stool samples, and how to take care of their hemorrhoids and other anal problems. So they learn to talk about it matter-of-factly. You can, too.

Okay, back to the butt. The party line on websites that talk about sex techniques is that there is nothing in the rectum, because poop is stored up higher. It moves down only when you feel an urgent need to go to the bathroom.

Well, actually, the truth is different, but only a little different. There is a little poop in there occasionally, but it's no big deal in terms of health risk. So the good news is that lots of times there is just no mess at all. Moreover, the chance of an unwelcome encounter is even lower than one might expect because the prostate isn't far inside the canal.

While I'm at it, let me note that there is a lot of pleasure to be had, for women as well as men, just inside the anal opening, where there is even less risk of messy. In any case, I'm going to give you lots of advice on how to make the experience work for both of you in all kinds of situations.

First of all, gals, you'll be using a glove, or your finger will be inside a female condom. So you will not get any poop on your skin. Not that it's a disaster if you do: You can just take it off with a handy wipe. Hey, changing a baby's diaper is no fun, but those of you with kids and grandkids survived it.

That said, some people like to clean themselves inside as well as out before playing. Using rectal syringes or enemas can be useful. However you may find, after some experimenting, that they are not worth the trouble.

For this purpose you can buy little plastic bulb syringes. The small ones are called ear syringes; the bigger ones, rectal syringes.

To use one, squeeze the bulb, hold the tip in warm water and release the bulb to fill. Then put a little lube on the tip (we'll discuss the choice of lubes later), find the anal opening with your finger, slide the tip in, squeeze out the water, and slide the tip back out. Usually, you'll be doing this sitting on the toilet. Then you hold the water in for a little while - you can experiment with different lengths of time - and then poop it out. You can do this several times until things feel clean inside.

You can also buy a Fleet's enema in the drug store: get the plain, non-laxative kind. If you cannot find that, just empty the bottle, and refill it with plain water. Do not use the commercial enema liquid for this purpose to avoid any irritation and over-active guts.

This sounds like a good plan, but sometimes the water makes a mess rather than cleaning one up. While before the clean-up procedure, there may be a couple of firm chunks of poop - I know, this is getting pretty graphic - the internal bath leaves a gooey slurry behind.

Another downside to enemas is that they can stimulate the intestines. Just when you are settling down to some sensual play, your colon may get noisy and busy - not so sexy. Every body reacts differently. So do experiment to see which methods are best for you.

Buying intimate supplies such as the rectal syringes is really no big deal. Generally, the drug store clerk could not care less about what they ring up and put into a bag for you. For that matter, they may not have a clue what the supplies are for. And if you are really shy about making eye contact with the teenager behind the counter, you can buy syringes anonymously online.

However, occasionally, one does get to have a little fun - or whatever you choose to make of it. The last time I picked up a rectal syringe from the drug store shelf and carried it to the cash register, the thought crossed my mind that, if this were a gross-out movie starring Seth Rogen, there would be sure to be a price check on this via store-wide loudspeaker.

Sure enough, the checker could not scan my purchase and did not know the price. And yes, she did get on the loudspeaker and called for a price check. And the guy at the back of the store did ask via the loudspeaker, "Price check on what?"

The clerk looked at me; I looked at her. We were both trying to decide whether to be embarrassed or tickled. I just cracked up, so she did, too.

Finally, I solved the problem by going back to the shelf and checking the price. So, in situations like this, you can either laugh or you can be embarrassed. And laughing is more fun. Usually, other people - in particular, your partner - will take their cues from you.

Another way to get squeaky clean inside is by performing the full-fledged enema routine, which ends in the evacuation of your colon as well as your rectum. That's a bigger project with the hoses and clamps and all that stuff. But some people enjoy it. So if you are one of them, go for it. Just one problem with either a rectal clean-up or an enema: both can lead to mild intestinal cramping before the deed is done.

The basics that make for a successful anal and prostate massage session are pretty straightforward. One is timing. After a good poop, you say, "Hey honey! I'm ready." This, by the way, is a great time for a quickie, if there is not enough time for a long session.

Another option is a self-check in the bathroom. You put on a glove, put lube or saliva on a finger as you are sitting on the toilet, then slide your finger into your anal opening and check on conditions inside. If the coast is clear, that can be very reassuring. If you find some stuff you'd rather not have there, it can sometimes be pooped out right then. The lube on the anus can help get the job done in a tidy manner.

I know, I know. This is way too much information with too much graphic detail. You really did not want to hear about your insides in such detail, did you? But it's time to get past this sort of thinking.

The alternative is to settle for less adventure - and less fun. And you don't want that!

Another easy way to go, if there is just too much in there and it is too messy to contemplate, is to skip the deep penetration part. This may be the time to just play with external anal massage and, maybe, add a little teasing with a fingertip inside the anal sphincter.

So, what happens if you do have a close encounter with the second kind? There's "full speed ahead and damn the torpedoes" approach (pun not intended, but I'll take a smile wherever I can get one). If you are in the mood for prostate massage and your partner is too, don't waste the opportunity. It is fine to just get in there and deal with what you find.

Here we go again with the graphic bits. There are ways to work around any obstacles that you may encounter. Once your finger is inside, if you feel some stuff in there, just slide your finger along the front wall of the rectum and ignore it. If there is matter up higher, just ignore it, too. You can even push little solid chunks further up out and out of the way.

Once you are done inside and slide your fingers out, you can hold on to the cuff of the glove with your pristine ungloved hand and pull the cuff towards the body as you are pulling your hand out. That way the glove turns itself inside out. Then, after you use a disposable wipe on him, tuck it into the used glove, tie the cuff into a knot and presto: all is tidy and ready for disposal. And no smell either.

It is a good general practice to always use a disposable wipe on his anus every time, and to not tell him whether this was a squeaky clean day or a not completely clean day. All he needs to know is that he had a great time. And that you, his partner, provided a really hot treat for him. Right?

And, in case you thought I wouldn't get around to this, here's another perspective on the messiness issue. In a recent phone conversation with Annie Sprinkle, the performance artist and sex educator who wrote the wonderful book, Spectacular Sex, she shared another possibility. "Some people" she explained, "find a bit of messiness a turn-on."

So there you are. If you are one of those people, or feel that you have the potential to become one, I am not going to judge you.

Finally, remember what your mama told you. Eat your high fiber diet to keep yourself regular. And a really, really basic piece of advice that we all tend to ignore: when nature calls, answer promptly. We tend to hold it and wait to go until the time is convenient. But you'll have more complete poops if you listen to your body and respect its signals.

There you are: the gross-out is over. Now sit back and read on to make the most of an organ you've been ignoring forever.

Genital Massage

Actually before we get to the prostate, let's talk a bit about massaging a body part that you are more familiar with. A genital massage for the guy (with or without a go at the prostate) is such an easy way for a couple to have fun by making him very happy.

So how is a genital massage different from a hand job? Well, in many ways they are similar because both involve the partner's hands on the man's penis and scrotum. However, the goal is a little different.

With a genital massage, the focus is on making the pleasure last. The point is not just to get him off, but to let him experience peaks and valleys along the way which is something most women understand from their own experiences. The idea is not to tease him but to allow him to enjoy himself longer. And also to experience a variety of sensations that are different from the joys of a simple hand job.

Receiving a genital massage can be a very nurturing experience, as well as fun, for a man. Check out the chapter on the long prostate massage session for information on how to organize the beginning of the genital massage. When the woman uses her hands to give him pleasure this way, she is starting to get him used to the idea of being done. He gets to experience what it is like when she is in charge and when he does not have to worry about being in charge. This can be a new experience for men, one that can be wonderful or difficult or both at the same time.

In our society, there is constant pressure on men to perform in the sexual arena, as well as everywhere else in daily life. Men are expected to change the flat tire and to deal with scary noises at night. Yes, this is a stereotype, and not every man feels that obligation and not every relationship works this way. But it is true much of the time.

Likewise, it is often the man who is expected to initiate sex: to turn her on, produce and maintain an erection, give her an orgasm, and to ejaculate (but not too early or too late). What's more, he is supposed to do the physical work of sexual intercourse - which by the way, gals - is a lot of work.

When he is getting a genital massage, there is no pressure to perform. All he needs to do is lie back and enjoy. Also, he doesn't have to fear doing anything wrong because he is the one who is being done and any reactions are okay.

Men also often worry whether they'll get an erection. But here that doesn't matter, which can be a big relief for the guy. So a genital massage is also a great choice to give sexual pleasure to a man when his erection is not happening, for whatever reason (which we all know happens to every man, more or less often.)

Men may also feel pressure to last longer before coming or, for that matter, not to come too late and tire her out. Or they may feel the need to come for her sake when they might actually prefer not to ejaculate this time around. But with genital massage, that does not matter either. It feels so lovely just to be the recipient of a loving touch.

Whether or not the erotic session will progress further to anal play and to prostate stimulation, it's always best to start each session with genital massage for him. It's also important to keep the sensations on the penis going when focusing on other areas such as the perineum and the anus.

So here's my advice for genital massage. Coat both your hands with lots of lube. Silicone lubricant is best for this because it does not dry out. Oil, such as coconut oil, also works well but may cause a latex glove to break. If you choose a water-based lube, have some water handy - a glass you can dip your fingers into or a spray bottle - to refresh the lube when it gets sticky.

The goal is to produce a continuous swirling motion over the head and the shaft of the penis, with lots of variations. You can use light touch like just the fingertips barely touching, all the way to firm touch like the whole palm grasping firmly or squeezing. The speed can also vary from so slow that you are barely moving to rapid strokes.

Do try different things and ask him if he likes them. Use yes or no questions; they take less thinking to answer, so that he can stay in that aroused happy state more easily. Ask him to show you what he likes by demonstrating on himself with his own hand. Now, since he may be self-conscious about doing that while you are watching, you may want to encourage him by telling him that it is a turn-on for you when he touches himself. Remember that what he likes for extended pleasure and what he likes to get to an ejaculatory orgasm may be different. So use your touch accordingly, depending on the goal that you both have in mind.

Here are some techniques for male genital massage. Grasp the shaft of the penis in the palm of your hand and slide up towards the tip, then back down. Use more pressure when going out towards the tip and less when moving towards the base of the penis. In fact, this is always a good guideline during genital massage. You always want to apply more pressure going towards the head of the penis than away from it to ensure that you don't bend the penis by mistake.

And while you're at it, you can add a twisting motion so that the hand slides around the penis while going up and down. You can also continue further up over the tip of the penis and slide the hand over the head of the penis and back down. Or you can roll the shaft between the palms of both hands, as if rolling a stick to make fire.

Also, both hands can follow each other sliding from the base to the head of the penis, but only sliding up. Another trick to try: with both hands on the shaft, gently slide them back and forth in opposite directions. You can vary the sensation of the strokes to make ejaculation less likely. And you can slow down - sometimes way down - to keep him from coming.

Of course you do not want to ignore the scrotum. There, the preferred sensations vary a lot. Some actually like their testicles squeezed a bit; others, not at all.

Most men, however, do love the sensation of swirling strokes on the scrotum. They may even like the skin pulled a little bit or to have it tickled. Now, as you've probably already noticed, the testicles tend to retract closer to the body just before his ejaculatory orgasm. And that is very useful information for the masseuse.

One last way to thrill him: Make a ring out of your pointer finger and thumb that encircles the scrotum, so that the testicles are just outside and the skin of the scrotum is snug over the testicles. Then tickle them with very light finger tips.

To make him come, you can use more repetitive motions on the penis the way he likes it. But do keep in mind that the trip is more than half the fun. Don't rush to the destination.

External Prostate Massage

Now for external prostate massage. This is a really important section, because your guy might say to you, "Yeah, I guess this prostate stuff is good for me, alright. So, you can do it. But just don't go anywhere near my butt." Lots of guys feel that way, especially at the beginning of the exploration.

Internal and external massage are not really equivalent. First, for someone who is having medical symptoms of prostatitis, external massage is just not effective. Thus a physician will always use internal massage to get the desired results. Second, the sensations from external massage will not be nearly as intense as direct prostatic massage, and the quality of the sensation is different. So think about external massage as a way station to internal massage.

But happily, there is still quite a lot that you can do for your guy on the outside. And yes, there is a lot of pleasure to be had with external prostate massage. Plus, it is easy to locate the right spot and easy to do. The bottom line is that he tells you what he likes. Then you try different ways of touching while asking him, "Do you like that?"

Guys, don't be shy (or disappointed) if you need to repeat that information for several sessions. It's not because she doesn't care, but because learning about you is so new to her.

The perineum, the sensitive spot, is located between the scrotum and the anus. It is a flat area between the thighs, sometimes referred to as the "taint" because "it ain't" the front and "it ain't" the back.

Women, as well as men, have a perineum. But the area is especially sensitive in men because the root of the penis continues there. You can feel it when the penis is erect. Remember to add the perineum to your genital massage repertory.

Here area some nice moves for the perineum: caress it lightly at first - just tickle it with your fingertips, with no lube. Start at the crack of the butt, ending with the scrotum. Then very slowly, progress to firmer pressure.

On the perineum, feel for the bony 'V' which points towards his front; it is right in the spot where the thighs meet the body. This is the location where firm touch can be felt in the prostate, although the latter is quite a way higher inside. Then apply mild to medium pressure with a pad of a finger inside the tip of the 'V'. You can pulse the touch, making small circles in the area. You can also use the entire length of two to three fingers to apply steady pressure over a larger area. Try mild-to-medium pressure that way, too.

This maneuver can feel really good to your guy during genital massage, and also during sexual intercourse and oral sex. It can also slow him down and help delay ejaculation.

You can massage the perineum with lube to create different sensations. Slowly caress the area with the pads of two or three fingers, very gently stretching the skin over the underlying tissues. Remember to vary mild to medium pressure, use small movements and go very slowly.

It feels good to him to pulse the perineum with the flat part of your fist or with the heel of your hand. Start with subtle vibrations, and then increase the intensity just a little at a time.

And do try a vibrator there - some guys go wild with that. Start with the lowest setting; if the vibrations are still too intense, use a fold or two of towel between the vibrator and the skin. And here is some motivation for the guy to keep experimenting: many men say that they can feel the exterior sensations more intensely and more pleasurably once they know the feelings from the interior prostatic massage.

External Anal Massage

Like it or not, your butt really is part of your life, actually a very important part of your life. Do you think we're spending too much time talking about your butt? What's the fuss?

Truth is, it's the site of a lot of health problems. Many of my patients seek medical help for a host of conditions related to the anus. And just like the prostate, the butt appreciates loving care so pay some attention to it and keep it healthy.

But I'm getting off track. We're here to talk about orgasms, not illness. And for the adventurous, the anal area offers a lot to like. It does not take a lot of energy or exertion to produce a ton of pleasure. Remember, too, the butt is an equal opportunity area: the techniques are really nice on women, too.

However, from now on, you'll need to keep your hands separate: one hand on the butt, one on the penis or on the vagina, so you don't mix the germs.

Moreover, it is better not to let your hands touch each other or a common surface. So if the penis hand picks up the lube bottle or pumps the handle, it's hands off for the butt hand.

Again, when you start working on his anal area, keep the genital stimulation going with the other hand, or with your mouth.

If he does not want to do more involved anal play, you can always just offer a super-light touch to the buttock area and a nice bun massage. They feel so yummy and are a lot more comfortable to start with. Actually, this applies whether or not the game is to grow more intimate. So begin with a feathery touch, one so light there is almost no contact. Then proceed to a firmer touch.

The light caresses are most intense before there is any other sensation. Just play - there is no goal except your pleasure. And the light tickle is really, really fun at the very top of the ass crack on the tiny hairs there and also over the buns. Make sure you take a long time here, especially if it is the first time and if there are hesitations about anal play.

Now onto the bun massage. Here you can use a fair amount of force, provided, of course, your partner approves. The gluteus muscles in the buns are big and strong, and are prone to holding tension. You can put your hands on either side of his hips and jiggle the buns back and forth, so they do the jello thing. You can make the buns jiggle in the same direction by holding on to the edges and wiggling them, or you can wiggle them in opposite directions so that they "kiss" over the anal opening. It looks really silly and feels really great.

Then you can just grab a bun in each hand - as much as you can hold - and squeeze, repeating in a slightly different place. You can also place one hand on each bun and knead in bread-dough fashion. Remember to watch your finger nails with all this.

Do all the bun stuff again using massage oil or lotion for totally different slippery sensations. Any of this bun play - the light caresses, the jiggling, the kneading - can be a great thing to do by itself, as a really good agenda for a quickie. And for an even quicker quickie, you can do it all with dry hands. Or you can start with dry hands and then use oil or lotion for the bun part.

When you are both ready for more, here's how you massage the anal opening. First put on a glove. You might want to start with just the one hand. But eventually, you'll want to use both, so keep extra gloves handy. Then take a long time to caress the outside of the anal opening lightly. Again, make the touch so very light that it hardly feels like touching at all. Often the most intense response comes before there is any firmer touch.

Just tickle with no lube, and be sure to reassure your partner that you'll not be going inside without asking first. That way, they can really relax and enjoy the great sensations. And do move slowly.

That may be as far as he wants to go, and that's just fine. However, if your partner wants more, put lube on your gloved fingers and caress slowly and lightly. Here's the most important part: pay close attention to what your fingers are feeling.

Let your finger do the walking, millimeter-by-millimeter, as you explore the skin at the anal opening. Remember that the one of you receiving this external anal massage is feeling tons of sensations through the millions of nerve ending there. Even though it may not look like a lot is happening, you can be sure it is having a fab impact.

Some specific moves to try:

Start in the middle of the anus, slowly stroking outward with the tip of one finger. Then reverse, stroking from the outside toward the center. You can put the pad of your finger on the anal opening closer in or further out and make lighter or firmer circles all around the opening. Just remember: slower is better.

Flatten your hand, then you put the little finger side along the ass crack. Using lots of lube, slide it up and down, letting each bump on the edge of the hand push a little into the anal opening. Just a tease; nothing more.

Take one thumb and slide it down the ass crack over the anal opening and a little bit further. Then take the other thumb and have it follow the first one. Keep that going like a roundabout for continuous sensation.

Tickle the anus with the tip of a butt plug or a dildo for a different sensation. For real intensity, you can also use a vibrator.

During this focus on anal play his erections may decrease for a while, which is totally normal. Erections will come and go, and that's fine. When his penis is soft, that doesn't mean he is not happy. It just means his focus is elsewhere.

External anal massage may keep both of you satisfied - even challenged - for months before you move on to the exploration of the inside. Or you may find that a few minutes of it has the lucky recipient begging for an internal massage. And it will be different on different days. Just remember the idea is to have fun and make connection, not to meet a predetermined goal.

Getting Inside

Why all this fuss about getting inside? Why a whole chapter on it?

Think about why you have been hesitant to experiment with this kind of sex. Probably, you were concerned about messiness, discomfort or even pain. And rightly so since it does take some knowledge about techniques (though nothing complicated) to avoid discomfort.

The whole process should always be pleasurable, or at least comfortable. Otherwise something is wrong and you need to stop right away. Or try something different or wait for another time.

When you have something, like a finger or a toy, in your butt, it is normal to have the unsettling feeling of needing to poop. But as you get used to anal play and realize the message is misleading, you'll learn to relax about that.

In a medical office like mine, doctors do internal anal exams by using a little lube and asking patients to bear down as if they were having a bowel movement. Then they slide the finger in, do the checking quickly and get back out. And they just hope that it wasn't too uncomfortable for the patient.

However, when you are with your partner, the priorities are very different. The idea is to have fun, and that means you should take a lot of time. You can also make sure that he is turned on by giving him genital pleasure. And before entering, you also make sure that he is warmed up with plenty of external anal play.

For some, the external anal stimulation takes only a few minutes before your partner is ready for more, as in, "Please baby. I've been waiting for this all my life." Or he may feel differently; it might take years before he wants you to enter him. Both are fine and normal.

Going inside the butt requires care and attention on the part of both partners, so it is important not to be drunk or high. If it is normal for you to have a glass of wine, that may be okay. However, if you aren't sober, there's the risk of emotional upset later, of doing too much too soon and then regretting it. Also if you are not paying close attention, there is a risk of harm to the anal area.

You never, ever want to force anything, either emotionally or physically. If you need to be drunk to be willing to try anal play, just don't do it. Sometimes, people use drugs like poppers to try to get the anal sphincters to relax. That is a really bad idea. It is much better to take more time, until he has learned to consciously relax those muscles. Until he can do that, what's the point of rushing? This is supposed to be fun.

Also don't ever use numbing creams or gels that are often employed to slow down ejaculation. If your body feels pain, you definitely do not want to mask it. You just need to listen to your body, and to keep your common sense engaged.

If your partner is truly ready, here's how to enter. First, put on a glove. And you use lots of lube because, unlike the vagina, the anal canal does not produce any lubrication.

Remember, too, that you can use band-aids over the fingertips or cotton balls inside the fingers of the glove to avoid giving discomfort. This works really well for just going inside. But you can't feel much with your fingertips covered. So once you actually get to the stage of massaging the prostate, you won't want to cover your fingertips. Short fingernails are ideal, but usually they do not have to be super-short.

Remember to keep the penis stimulation going the whole time and to watch him closely. Is he holding his breath? Is he catching his breath? Do you hear a little gasp? All three are signals to slow down. Also watch his face for reactions. The breathing part, by the way, applies to you as well as your partner.

Back up for a moment. You have one hand on his penis and one hand on his butt. Then you ask, "May I go in?" and wait for an answer. This is really, really important. Don't ever surprise him. Provide him with warning, as well as with a chance to say no. If he does say yes, still take your time and go in slowly.

The funny thing is that, very often it is difficult to tell for sure where the anal opening is. So it is totally okay to put your finger in one spot and ask, "Is this the right place?" Then request that he push down, as if he were having a bowel movement to help him relax his sphincter muscle. Now you press in with your finger tip, as if you were ringing a door bell. Push a tiny bit and stop, giving you both time to get acquainted. When you feel the muscle relaxing, gently push in a bit further. Just this much is bound to be exciting. You really don't need to rush in at all.

At this point if he says "stop," don't remove your finger abruptly, that is too startling. Simply stop moving and then slowly slide out. If he does not like your finger inside, then revert to gentle external massage and wait for another day.

Going inside him can be emotional for the guy. It can be arousing, it can be pleasurable, or it can be sort of just neutral. And if the gal is on the receiving end, the same possibilities apply. It can be an emotional experience, exciting and/or pleasurable. Or it could be not much of anything.

However, for the gal who is doing the finger inside the guy, it can be really exciting for her to be the one who is penetrating. When everything's working, everybody wins.

ERIKA THOST MD

Internal Anal Massage

Now so some tips on technique. And gals, share these notes with your guys, because what's fun for men turns out to be fun for women too, even if they don't have prostates.

As a general rule, use super-slow motions because even tiny movements create lots of sensation. In fact, movements should be so slow that the woman who is giving the massage will almost be bored. Well, not really; doing this massage is a big turn-on for most of us. You really won't have to do much to make him very, very happy.

While massaging, pay close attention to his face for clues as to how he is doing. Keep breathing and keep the genital stimulation going. Now, as with external massage, it's normal for erections to come and go. And again, let me emphasize that the loss of his erection doesn't mean he isn't enjoying himself.

It just means that he is focused elsewhere in his body.

At first you go in no deeper than the fingertip if that's what he wants. If he's up for it, you can try pushing your fingertip to the side, to the front, to the other side and back (needless to say, really slowly). This is with your fingertip just barely inside him.

You can do the same thing moving in very slow circles just inside the anal opening. Go easy on the in-and-out motions since they can cause soreness if overdone.

You might want to try some slow movements in and out with a super slow corkscrew twisting motion, which is very cool, however you'll want lots of lube for that. In later sessions you might try more of those in-and-out movements if he likes them. And yes, keep asking him what he likes.

Do use lots of lube on his penis as well as on his anus. If the water-based lube gets sticky, dip your finger in water. Or if you are using silicone, just add a little more. And for a super-slippery experience, mix some silicone-based lube with some water-based lube; it's a wonderful combination.

You may have heard that you can't use too much lube, but that's not quite right. You don't want to get a whole lot of silicone lube inside the butt because silicone is never absorbed. So it just sits there, and can leak out later, which is not a disaster, but not precisely what you want to be doing at the office or the dinner table. Water-based lube does not cause this problem.

Here is where, instead of a glove, you might want to try a female condom. Usually you'll take out the internal ring for this and throw it away or save it to use for Christmas tree ornaments. Just kidding! Then put your fingers inside the condom, slide it inside him, and move your finger inside it. The condom itself doesn't move, just your finger. This provides even greater insurance against messy.

One important thought: if he is really aroused and asks you to do him hard, be careful. If he is really turned on, his pain tolerance is going to be higher than normal and he may end up being sore afterwards. You can always be more intense the next time.

ERIKA THOST MD

Prostate Massage

You've arrived at the most exciting part of the course. The suspense probably just about killed you, didn't it? It is surprising to most people how much learning and prep work are needed to assure a fabulous experience.

I should mention that when a physician like myself does a prostate massage, it is, of course, not meant to be arousing. The massage may be very effective as therapy for prostate problems. However, sexual arousal is not part of the experience. You have the advantage of doing it with a sexual partner, so that you get to have the erotic as well as the health benefits. And the sexual turn-on certainly makes prostatic massage much more pleasurable.

Back to technique. To massage the prostate, use lots of lube. If the lube isn't dripping off the ceiling, it's not enough.

To help you find the location of the prostate, remember that it is on the penis side of the rectum. I know that sounds silly, but it's actually useful to recall that when he is in different positions.

Once inside, slide your finger up the front, his belly side. If he is on his back, that means that the flat of your finger is pointing to the ceiling.

Be sure to use the pad of your finger. Do not use the actual fingertip, because it pokes. This is really important: you want to pay attention to make sure that the flat side of your finger is on the prostate.

You'll probably find that the pointer finger of your dominant hand works best. Since it does not have another finger on both sides, there is a little more mobility. Some people like using a middle finger because it is longest and provides the most reach. It is worth trying both to see what works best for you both.

So you slide your finger up a couple of inches and feel a firm flat round disc and that's it. You've found the Holy Grail! Exciting, isn't it?

The prostate may feel like a chestnut, a coin or a half of a walnut. It has a round-to-oval shape with two lobes like the wings of the butterfly. There is some tissue between your finger and the prostate which can vary in thickness. Sometimes the prostate is right there at your fingertips, and sometimes you can feel more of that soft tissue in-between.

You might be able to feel his pulse just like you would at the wrist or at the neck. As your finger rests on his G-spot you can feel the rhythm of his heartbeat. Cool, isn't it! And so intimate!

At first just hold a little light pressure with your finger tip without moving. Then start to touch the prostate so very lightly that it can be hard to tell whether you are actually touching or not. Keep it that light for a while - there is no rush to get anywhere else. Never do fast and hard movements right on the prostate. And do keep the genital massage going.

He should feel free to say "enough" at any time. Your task is to listen and to respond, sliding your finger out promptly but not rapidly.

This prostate massage may feel good to him, or it may just feel "interesting". It usually feels more pleasurable after he has experienced it more often. Here's a surprising finding: even if the prostate massage does not feel that good to him yet, his ejaculatory orgasm will still be more intense with greater volume. So he may get the benefit of the deeper orgasms before he notices pleasurable sensations in the prostate itself.

Do you both want more? Are you both ready for the actual "massage" part of the prostate massage? Here the focus is not on moving in and out; you move while staying inside. And you avoid any hard or fast movements directly on the prostate.

During the massage, the guy usually cannot tell exactly what the woman is doing with her finger on his prostate. The sensations tend to be diffused. So don't bother writing messages to him by tracing letters with your fingers on his prostate. He won't be able to decipher them.

There are a bunch of good massage moves. One is called "windshield wipers": your fingertip slowly moves back and forth over his prostate while your hand remains stationary. Another is to trace circles right on the prostate. Yet another is to do strokes from the edges in towards the middle and from top to bottom. With therapeutic prostate massage, these moves are designed to drain the fluid that collects in the prostate.

You can do light pulses by gently pushing into the prostate and then letting go. With the "come hither" motion, you bend your finger and stroke the prostate as if you were beckoning to someone. Last, there is the "trip around the world" in which you slide your finger circularly around the edges of the prostate.

As I described in the positions section, you may need to lean way in there to go deep inside him. Don't worry if you cannot touch the whole thing. Just stroke what you can reach. The far edge is especially difficult to reach unless your fingers are long.

During prostate massage (and this applies to anal and genital massage, too) your partner may feel unexpected emotions - love or laughter, fear or anger, sadness or tears. It can also be a mixture of these feelings. Don't worry, this is normal and desirable. You just keep the massage going, letting the feelings happen. You do not need to say or fix anything.

Do occasionally ask him, "Do you like this?" Use "yes or no" questions so that he does not have to think, so that he can stay in a state of relaxed arousal. Keep the penis stimulation going the whole time to help keep him happy.

Now here is a very exciting part: the "fireworks finale" to prostate massage, which very few people in the whole world have experienced. So few, that you almost never hear anyone talk about their experience with the prostate during ejaculation.

The first time this occurred with my husband, my thoughts were, "Wow! What was that? Did that really happen?" The second time was a few months later - after all, one doesn't tend to do these things every day. And yes! It really did happen again.

I felt I had discovered something totally new: undiscovered territory on the world map. It is so amazing to go to medical school and think you know pretty much all there is to know about the human body. What a surprise to find the body right in front of me doing something that I had never even heard of.

Here's what I'm talking about. If you have your finger on the prostate and the man is about to ejaculate, the prostate poofs out and gets firmer. And then, as he is ejaculating, it shrinks back to normal. There is no pulsing. It is just a one-time thing of it getting big and then contracting back.

Amazing, isn't it! This gland that we thought just sits there, calm and inscrutable, is actually is quite busy during ejaculation.

The puffing out of the prostate happens at the same time he is experiencing that feeling of inevitability, that feeling of "Oh! I'm gonna come." So in a sense, he has a way of communicating his ecstasy without making a sound. Experiencing his orgasm this way is very intimate and exciting. I think it's the best show on earth!

By the way, the finger communication is just one way of finishing the fabulous experience. You may choose to go from the prostate massage to sexual intercourse before he orgasms. Nothing wrong (and a lot right) with that!

ERIKA THOST MD

Prostate Milking

There are several slightly different definitions of the term prostate milking. Some people find the term 'prostate milking' more erotic than prostate massage even though the terms mean essentially the same thing.

Prostate milking is massaging the prostate with the aim of expelling seminal fluid from the prostate through the penis. This happens without an ejaculatory orgasm. Prostate milking is the same thing as prostate massage. However some men (and their givers) like the idea of expelling some fluid during that massage which is not part of the ejaculation.

The idea is to 'clean out' the gland. It also stimulates blood flow. This can be for the purposes of pleasure or for prostate health benefits, or both.

The fluid can be a few drops or more. Many men find that idea exciting and appealing however it is really not all that common to get fluid, especially a lot of fluid.

There is often a component of fantasy in the concept of prostate milking. It can be a great fantasy to get the prostate stimulated and have fluid released. Sometimes this includes being dominated. It is just fine to have fun with this erotic desire. If you choose to act out this fantasy, just make sure that the actual prostate massage is still done with gentleness and awareness.

To milk the prostate you use the same techniques that we have discussed at length in the rest of this course. The motion most conducive to prostate milking are smooth, gentle, continuous strokes from the top to the bottom of the prostate. There can be stimulation of the penis with hand or mouth at the same time, or not.

Doctors will use what they call 'prostate massage' to get fluid to use in diagnosis. This the same thing that others may call prostate milking.

So have a great time exploring prostate milking as another aspect of prostate massage!

Putting It All Together

We've covered how to do all the stages: external prostate, external anal, getting inside, internal anal, and prostate massage. This chapter is about how to put all that together for one fun session.

Remember there are really no rules other than safety and mutual consent. This session is for you both to play in any way that the two of you want. It's great if this turns out to be hot and sexy. And it's certainly okay if it turns out to be an adventure, a walk on the wild side.

That said, here's a map for putting it altogether. The guy may wish to go to the bathroom to check himself as we talked about in the messy section. He might want to take a quick shower, or maybe use handy wipes for that, instead. Now you want to warm up the room so you are both comfortable without clothes and gather all your supplies.

When you start, take a second to be with each other. Maybe share some kisses. And guys, don't forget to get her turned on, too. Maybe the two of you want some regular sexual play first, whatever that is for you. Maybe some oral sex for her, some clitoral stimulation, maybe a little vibrator action, maybe some G-spot massage. She may want to have some orgasms, or to save them for later.

Next, position him comfortably. And tell him that this is a treat meant just for him in three different ways. First, remind him that he does not have to do anything, other than lie there and enjoy, but that he is still totally in charge. He can request things, he can say yes or no to anything. Second, tell him that having an erection is fine, not having one is fine, and anything in between is fine too. And third, tell him that he is free to ejaculate early, or in the middle, or late, or never. Whatever he wants.

After that you might want to express appreciation of his penis and his ass. Tell him how handsome and sexy he looks. Keep your eyes on him. He may want to look at you, or just close his eyes and let the sensations wash over him.

Start with just general body touch, caressing and stroking everywhere to wake up his senses. Then a bun massage - a firm and deep one - would hit the spot. The next step is a genital massage, which you keep going during the whole session. Maybe some oral sex on him and maybe some nipple stimulation if he likes that sort of thing. And I do realize that you'll run out of hands somewhere along the way.

Next on the agenda is the external anal massage. Remember, as always, that it is really, really important to ask - and wait for his answer - before going inside. Then slide in your finger, do an internal anal massage, and the actual prostate massage. Keep asking him what he likes, phrasing the questions for yes or no answers.

And also remember that, during the genital, anal and prostate massage, emotions may come up for him, just like they might for a woman during a G-spot massage. These feelings are unrelated to the fun task at hand. They're about him, not you. They are just old, diffused emotions that he is releasing. Don't ask him about them or add comments, other than maybe to say, "You are doing great."

He may end up having the experience of some non-ejaculatory orgasms, some peaks of sensation. Maybe he will want to have an orgasm towards the end. Maybe he'll want to use his own hand for that, with your help or with you just watching. If your fingers are inside him, they may exit slowly or stay put; his choice.

Men like varying amounts of sensations on the penis as an orgasm finishes. So you'll need to learn that about him. Some guys get a huge kick out of having your finger on the prostate at that moment, and some really don't.

Remember, too, that a successful session may end with no orgasm. He may have had enough, or maybe your hand is tired, or maybe it's time for you to have another orgasm, or whatever. You may end up having intercourse.

After sliding out, hold the back of your hand or your fist against the outside of his anal opening for a few moments, so he doesn't feel lonely. This parting can be a very emotional experience akin to parting from a lover. On the other hand, some guys don't care about that at all.

You do a quick bit of cleanup with handy wipes. And then it is nice to appreciate each other, to thank each other. Tell him that you loved doing that, that it was hot for you. Tell her that you loved getting it, that you felt loved. Then you may cuddle. He may want to sleep a little. Don't make him feel guilty about that. He's done a great job of exploring, and you've done a great job exploring with him.

And there you are - that's all there is to it. The only really important take-away is to have the courage to explore your sexuality at this new level.

ERIKA THOST MD

Love Those Quickies!

This book is mostly about slow play. But quickies can be great, too! Truth is, a quickie is sometimes all there's time for. If you don't take advantage of these brief opportunities, you're going to miss out on a lot of sex, fun and connection.

Quickies are not second-best to the long love making sessions, either. They are just as wonderful in their own way if we let them be. Just like there are times when we love a plain old hamburger and fries and other times we crave a fancy bouillabaisse that has been lovingly prepared for hours.

In any case, it's just so much better to have a short lovemaking session than none at all. If you always wait for the perfect time to have sex, you're going spend a lot of time waiting. And actually, since quickies are by nature improvised and imperfect, you may find you're more relaxed and playful. There is less pressure to make the experience perfect, which may allow you to be more spontaneous and adventurous than usual. And that's what we want.

Remember, too, it can even be fun to just take a break from the belief that sex must end in orgasm. Start with some erotic play, and maybe the orgasm will happen and maybe not. And guys, you will have a lot more sex with your partner if she is just free to be sexy with you without feeling like she has to create that ejaculatory orgasm for you every time.

Of course, you want it a lot of the time and you will get it. But maybe orgasm doesn't have to be the ending every single time.

So here is the secret to making quickies happen: Whenever you feel the smallest erotic impulse, whenever you feel even a tiny bit of a turn on, jump at the chance. Even two minutes can be fun.

Perhaps the two of you lock yourselves in the bathroom, she drops on her knees, unzips his pants and pulls them down, gives him oral sex first for a few minutes and then adds external prostate massage for another few minutes. Then, time to go.

Okay, so that was more than two minutes. But it was still really short. She helps him get dressed, they kiss and go back to family life.

Maybe another time, our couple has seven spare minutes until they have to leave for dinner. She playfully pushes him down on the bed, sits on his face, and enjoys a few minutes of receiving oral sex. Then they finish getting dressed and leave. Oops: probably best if he washes his face.

With practice, his prostate can be incorporated, too. As he learns to relax and allow a finger into his anal opening, he can have a quickie prostate massage when he is in the mood. Maybe he is in the shower, and she joins him. She rubs conditioner on both hands, one hand caresses his genitals and the other caresses his butt. When he's ready, she slides a finger in, gives his prostate some gentle strokes for a few minutes and that's it. Both wash and step out of the shower with a special glow on their faces. Now that's a really good reason for checking out the guy's reaction to conditioner on his penis and anus ahead of time, isn't it?

For a full genital and prostate massage session, it's best to have about an hour. However, even 30 minutes can be enough for a mini-prostate massage, or at least for a genital massage and some external anal caresses to keep him in practice for enjoying that kind of caress from you.

So how do you make quickies work? The trick is to get yourself turned on while you're starting. Consciously, work on increasing your arousal while you collect your supplies. Think about the yummy feelings that you'll be having soon, and speak those juicy thoughts out loud to your partner. You might want to move your body in way that feels sexy to you. For women it might be arching your back, rolling your hips, rubbing your breasts against him even if you are still dressed. He might move his hips imagining how it feels to be inside her. Either one of you might think or speak an erotic fantasy. And don't worry about being a little silly; it's the thought that counts. Even if you laugh about it, you'll still get turned on.

Another time over dinner (with just the two of you) tell each other some sexy fantasies, so that later those stories can be told back to you to get you turned on. The idea is to be primed for arousal. But once you start touching each other, do keep the touch slow. Hectic foreplay just isn't sexy.

Gals, go for his penis (with your hand or mouth) to get him turned on fast. And play with letting his turn-on get you excited too.

Now here we are mostly talking about quickies for prostate massage. However, let's make sure that she is the prime beneficiary of her share of quickies and that you both set aside enough time for long sessions. And gals, make sure that you request these sessions, in a nice, enthusiastic and appreciative way.

If anal play is to be part of your quickie, use a handy wipe on his butt as a substitute for a shower. Then do the same things that you would in a long session, only for a shorter period. You do the genital massage, the external anal massage, the internal anal after asking and receiving permission to enter, and the prostate massage. To get inside him more quickly, he can take the initiative to tell her when he's ready. And he can focus on pushing out against her finger and then relaxing to make the process go faster.

When I do a prostate exam as a physician, it only takes a couple of minutes. So certainly, a few minutes is definitely possible, once he's entirely comfortable with the idea of being penetrated.

It's totally okay to end these sessions quickly, too. A look of gratitude, a kiss and appreciative "That was so hot!" should suffice. And use that bubbly energy left over from your quickie in whatever regular stuff you are doing that day. A quickie is really great for fueling creative thought: to write that next chapter or to get inspired to plant the garden.

Later on, it can be part of the fun to talk briefly about what parts of your sexy adventure worked well. Then file away the thoughts - or maybe write a diary entry on your computer - for future reference. Nothing says love quite so much as a surprise offer of a rerun of a sexy treat that he or she has especially enjoyed in the past.

Safety First

I have consulted with professional colleagues who are urological specialists and they are unanimous: they see no risk in prostate massage, except maybe from a long finger nail. Moreover, these colleagues think massage is likely to reduce current prostate symptoms and perhaps prevent future ones. I have also researched the medical literature via the Online Medical Search services and the brand new Campbell's Urology textbook. None contain cautions for prostatic massage. Research continues, however, and new and different information may develop. So do keep checking.

It is always really important that you pay attention to pain during the massage and back off right away. If any pain persists, or develops later, do see a physician. And also remember that this information here is only for inspiration: you really do need your own doctor for medical care.

For the man: do double-check with your doctor that prostate massage is safe for you. And do get regular checkups for sexually transmitted diseases and cancer by your doctor. There should not be any prostatic massage for about three weeks before a PSA test, the controversial test for prostate cancer. It may distort the results.

Keep in mind, too, some simple rules to assure safe sex. If you and your partner have both been tested and you are both monogamous, then you may consider yourselves "fluid bonded". And then you will probably need gloves only for cleanliness.

If you are with a new partner or you have not been tested, or if you are with multiple partners, gloves (or other barriers) are a must. Also be careful about sharing toys, and cover them with condoms too.

Be careful with handling lube bottles so you don't mix anal and genital germs. Clean up is easier if you put a condom on the lube bottle. However you still need to keep track of your hands so the same hand always touches the lube bottle.

While we're at it, make sure you only use toys in the butt that have a flared base so they can't slide in all the way. There are some websites that are good resources on safer sex issues, including San

Francisco Sex Information and Planned Parenthood websites. So please stay updated on the current recommendations.

ERIKA THOST MD

Supplies

Lots of the stuff you need for prostate massage is available at pretty much any drug store.

For online stores: their phone consultants are totally comfortable with questions about products ranging from butt plugs to special-purpose lubes, and they usually really know what they are talking about.

Go ahead and buy a fair amount of stuff. It really doesn't cost that much, and it really pays to experiment to find what works best for the two of you. For the price of a meal and a movie out you can collect treasures that will be a lot more rewarding than a steak dinner and a couple tickets to Die Hard 27.

Handy wipes come in very handy, indeed. You'll want to try both the scented and unscented kind. Some people really like the scented sort; the pretty smell makes them more comfortable. But watch for skin reactions.

And gloves, of course, are very important. So make sure you try different kinds to see which feel right for you. They come in latex, vinyl, and nitrile. And they come in a variety of sizes. The one-size-fits-all are okay but not best. And when you are choosing sizes, better to go too big than too small. If you are nervous and your hands are perspiring, it's easier to get on a glove that's not too snug. One other thought: Try the silly and sexy black gloves that you can find online.

The other thing you may want to get is female condoms. They come in boxes, so they're not usually on the drugstore racks with the male condoms. Instead they tend to be on a shelf, mixed in with pregnancy kits and the like. They can be hard to find in stores so best shop online at sites including Amazon, where they are easy to locate and cost a bit less.

People often use finger cots, mini-condoms that fit on the finger-tip, for anal play. I don't recommend them because they cover too little, which will either inhibit your play or risk a mess.

You might want to try some cotton balls or some band aids in your gloves. As I mentioned earlier, they are kinder to his insides, eliminating the possibility of poking or pinching. The catch is that they also reduce feeling in the fingertips, making it harder to know what you're touching and reducing the sense of intimacy with your partner. You two need to decide whether the cushioning is worth it.

Interestingly, though, a lot of women find that they enjoy having a finger inside the anus more if there is something to pad the fingernail. So maybe the best thing is to try it both ways before choosing.

Now for the all-important lubes. Drug stores and similar shops usually carry lots of brands of water-based lubes. But do read the label before you buy. The scented and flavored lubes never work, other than to irritate the delicate tissues, just skip them.

One lube that I think is really great is silicone lube - pure silicone - and you can always tell you are getting the real thing by the high price: a little bottle costs more than $20. The good news is that a little goes a long way. You're not going to need much because it does not dry out once exposed to the air, like water-based lubes. A popular brand is called Pjur Eros, the black bottle. Your local or online adult store sells it.

Best to try different ones to see which you both like. Pump bottles are really great for lube because they are so handy.

Another thing you might want to buy at the drug store: disposable, absorbent water-proof pads for protecting sheets. The Chux brand is just fine. Make sure to buy the biggest size they have; nobody wants to be distracted by cleanup issues.

I mentioned using regular male condoms for butt toys. This makes sense for several reasons. The first is easy cleanup, all you need do is turn it inside out as you are pulling it off, and there you are. Second, if you are practicing safer sex with your partner and sharing toys, you need the protection. Lastly, if you have a silicone toy and are using silicone lube, direct contact between the two will wreck the toy. Non-lubricated condoms are great for toys because the toy will be dry and not slippery with lube when you remove the condom.

Stuff you probably already have: lots of pillows and cushions because you want to be really comfortable. Perhaps grab some towels to put underneath. And then you want a nice music source, preferably with a remote control (you'll both be busy...).

Music is really, really important, and many people use music that is too slow. They play some lovely meditative music, and then wonder why he goes to sleep. For better energy all round, find some music with a beat. Choose it together, as part of the adventure.

Then collect all your toys: the butt plugs, the vibrators, maybe some feathers for tickling and whatever else you've splurged on from your favorite neighborhood or online adult store. Have some water handy, some yummy juices, some snacks that you love to nibble. And of course you've got to have some chocolate. Milk chocolate or dark chocolate - your decision. However, I do believe very strongly that chocolate goes very beautifully with erotic play.

ERIKA THOST MD

Positions

Wondering about the best positions for doing prostate massage? The basic idea is to do whatever works. And depending on your age, physical condition and mood, that can mean anything from acrobatic to totally restful. But do try different positions to see what is comfortable, yet still provides room for variety and the full range of sensations.

Remember: the woman who is giving the massage needs to be comfortable too. If her back is killing her, everybody loses. She may want to lean against the head board or the wall. Or use a BackJack type floor chair, which is a sitting device that you find on the Web. She'll probably lean forward, anyway, once things get truly exciting because she may need to lean way in to go deep. But the back support is still good to have.

If the guy is on his back, which is nice because you can look at each other, you might want to put a pillow under his hips for better access. If he is on his side, there's a chance of losing your bearings on the landmarks. Just keep in mind that the prostate is on the penis side, on the front of his body.

Another position for the guy is on his tummy, which makes it is easy for him to close his eyes, zone out and just enjoy. The tricky part is there is less access to his genitals. Another nice position is on his hands and knees, or for the flexible in the crowd, on his hands and knees but sitting back on his heels.

One really, really key thing to remember: if you're not having fun, if things are not flowing, if something is just not quite right, or if you want things to be better, it's really great to move into a new position. It's amazing how big a difference that can make.

And then there is an issue of the massage table versus the bed. If you already have a massage table, try it. She might enjoy being able to stand up while she's playing. Or she can perch between his legs on the massage table. If you don't have one, I'm not sure it's worth buying one for just this purpose. A big bed, or even a towel on the carpet, really does work well because it gives you both more room to spread out.

Here's a technique for going deep inside him, to reach the top of his prostate. Position him on his back with you sitting on his right (assuming you're right-handed) alongside his belly. Then you bend forward and slide your right index finger inside him from between his thighs. You may end up bending forward so far that your shoulder is all the way down against the bed - in other words, with you lying on or kneeling over his right leg.

Another position is recommended while using the Aneros prostate massager which we will talk about in the next chapter. This position is on his side with both legs bent, the top leg bent more than the bottom. This, by the way, can also be a good for prostate massage without the Aneros.

ERIKA THOST MD

Sex Toys

Toys offer an easy way to add spice and pleasure to your sex life, both for men and women. The toys that concern us here are those meant for anal insertion and massage. All can be used with a partner or solo.

The insertion of toys may not be entirely pleasurable for some men right at the start, just as prostate massage may not feel good at first. Therefore, beginning anal play needs to be gentle and should be combined with genital pleasure to build the positive association for men.

You must be careful about one thing: do not insert any toy into the anus that lacks a flared base or other guard. Toys have a way of disappearing inside, possibly necessitating an embarrassing emergency room visit. Believe it or not, that happens all the time. If it happens to you, make things easy for everyone and just tell them the truth in the emergency room. They have seen it all, lots of times!

The primary types of sex toys for anal play are prostate massagers, butt plugs, dildos, and vibrating toys.

The Aneros prostate massagers and similar devices are getting rave reviews from many men. Their use is entirely hands-free, because they have little wings that stay outside and perch on the perineum. During prolonged play, you may need a washcloth to pad the wings if the pressure on the perineum is a bit too much.

The Aneros looks a little like a narrow asymmetric egg. At one end is a neck, with little wings that stick out sideways at the tip. To use it, apply lube and insert the egg-shaped part slowly and carefully. Once inside, the device stays in place very nicely, all by itself. To generate more intense pressure from the Aneros, contract your anal sphincter (the muscle you also use to stop the flow of urine). You can contract a little or a lot, and you can do the contractions slowly or fast.

The Aneros works well slipped inside while the man receives a genital massage - that is certainly a special treat. Also, some men enjoy having sexual intercourse with it in place. Then it works fine either with the man on the bottom or on top.

Regular butt plugs look like little cones with narrow necks and flared bases, designed so they will neither fall out nor get lost inside. They come in a bewildering variety of sizes, and it may be best to start really small and work up. Butt plugs are usually inserted and then left in the anus, rather than providing an in-and-out motion. Be careful to insert the toy slowly and gently (and remove it that way, too) for a maximum of pleasurable sensation. Butt plugs can pop out if the wearer moves a lot or bears down.

Dildos usually look like penises, more or less. However, some are designed to seem 'lifelike', and some are works of art, resembling animals, people, etc. They also vary a lot in size. For anal use, be sure to get one with a flared base so it cannot be sucked in. Dildos tend to pop out even more than butt plugs if not held in by a hand or clothing. Use them with a very gentle and very slow in-and-out motion and with lots of lube.

Dildos work well for anal play for both men and women since it's possible to start small and gradually increase the size of the dildo you are using. Better too small than too big for pleasurable first experiences. It's nice to have an array of sizes and shapes on hand so that the receiver can choose the one he's in the mood for.

A dildo can be used with a strap-on harness by women or men. The harness used can be traditional position, with the dildo located where a penis would be. This provides more of the look and feel of sexual intercourse. Alternatively, the harness can be wrapped around the thigh. This method is less tiring to the wearer of the harness, and actually provides for more precision of movement.

When planning to use a butt plug or dildo for anal play, it is best to cover it with a condom. Use a non-lubricated condom because it is less sticky, and put it on ahead of time so that you do not need to interrupt your play.

Condom use is especially important if you are using safer sex practices with your partner. But even if you do not need to use barriers for safety's sake, condoms make cleanup much easier. They also prevent discoloration and clinging odors.

The tricky part about shopping for sex toys is that there are zillions of them, ranging greatly in price, material and quality. So research and shop carefully. It is possible to spend a lot of money and end up with a closet full of sex toys that mostly go unused. Educate yourself before you buy.

Many toys are silicone or rubber-based (it should say on the packaging) and thus cannot be used with any greasy lube or oil, which damage the material. If you use a silicone sex toy, use only water-based lube. Or you can cover the toy with a condom and then use any lube.

Small butt plugs can be inserted entirely into a condom, flared base and all. For larger dildos, the condom is rolled onto the shaft, just as on a real penis.

There are also some sex toys that are meant to be hand-held, either by the man or by his partner. They clean up well in hot soapy water, so you may not wish to use a condom with them.

These toys are S-shaped or shaped like a honey-dipper. You hold them in your hand, slide them in, and vary the angle by applying pressure on the handle. It can be quite a bit of work to use these, but many people love them. If the active partner gets tired, you may prefer to switch to a toy that stays inside by itself.

You can also find some anal and prostate toys that vibrate. Again, make sure that they have flared bases so they can't vibrate their way too far inside the rectum. The jury is out on these toys: often, the vibration is too weak to make a difference, or is not in a good location to feel really great. There is huge variation of opinion on the benefit of these toys, due to anatomical differences as well as preferences in individual sensation. So you really just need to do some experimenting.

However, there is one vibrating sensation that most men like: the good old Hitachi vibrator that is so beloved by women. Hold in on his perineum, using a little hand towel between the vibrator and the skin to dampen the intensity at first. It can also be used directly on his penis.

Remember to use a lot of lube with any insertion toys. Sometimes it can be difficult to get the lube where it is really needed, which is on the inside the anal opening. One method is to coat the toy (or the condom that is covering the toy) with silicone lube first, and then use water-based lube after that.

Another way is to insert some lube before beginning with the toy. There is a device called a 'lube shooter' that is sold in sex shops; the Aneros company has a similar device called the Marksman. This is a blunt syringe, whose tip you carefully insert into the anal opening, and then push the plunger to slide a measured quantity of lube inside. Make the use of a lube inserter be part of playing, rather than just a preparation for play. And be sure to coat the butt plug or dildo with lube as well, even though there is already lube inside.

It is worth your while to do your research online to find and buy the items that will work for you. Have a good time researching online and trying things out in real life!

ERIKA THOST MD

Therapeutic Prostatic Massage

When therapeutic prostatic massage - also called TPM - is done by a doctor or other medical professional, there is nothing sexual about it. It is a purely medical procedure.

Why would a man come to a medical professional for a TPM? The purpose is both to prevent prostate problems and to treat prostate problems, such as Chronic Prostatitis and Benign Prostatic Hypertrophy.

TPM can help prevent prostate and pelvic problems since it promotes increased circulation and decreased muscle tension. TPM, just like prostate massage by partner, should not be done if there is any acute infection or any cancer.

There is a health issue that a few unlucky men have, called Chronic Prostatitis or Chronic Pelvic Pain Syndrome or Nonbacterial Prostatitis. This is pain in their pelvic area that does not resolve with antibiotics, like Acute Prostatitis does. Basically this is a general diagnosis for pain in the male pelvis that cannot be identified.

Chronic Prostatitis or chronic pelvic pain can be a really big problem in a man's life. The pain can be severe and constant. It does not help that in our society there is little awareness of this health problem, and therefore little sympathy. He really cannot talk about it anywhere. And there are no real solutions. Typically the urologist has tried different antibiotics already, and the antibiotics are not helping.

One treatment for male chronic pelvic pain is TPM, either by itself or in combination with antibiotics. And many men also utilize it on a regular basis after they improve to prevent recurrence. With TPM there is draining of the ducts plus increased circulation in the prostate. Also there is attention to the surrounding muscles and tendons to reduce inflammation and to relax the tissues as well as to increase the circulation. This can help to break the vicious cycle of tension in the pelvis which leads to pain which leads to more tension. TPM can provide immediate improvement in the symptoms as well as healing of the tissues in the long term.

Many men in their middle age and beyond have symptoms of BPH or Benign Prostatic Hypertrophy which is enlargement of the prostate, without cancer. These symptoms mainly are urinary difficulties such as weak stream, hesitancy, urgency, and frequency. It is also associated with erectile dysfunction, lower sexual desire and lower sexual satisfaction.

Typically men will see their urologist for BPH. There are several types of medication for it. One newly recommended medication for BPH is daily Cialis which is great because it helps with the symptoms and also helps increase sexual performance. TPM also helps with the symptoms of BPH to prevent them and improve them.

Just like a therapeutic body massage is non-sexual and makes you feel better, the therapeutic prostatic massage is non-sexual and makes the man feel better. It is so gratifying to see the patient walk out of the office with a lightness in his body and a spring in his step.

It takes place in a medical office, on an exam table, in a treatment room with bright lights and a clinical attitude. There is no touch at all to the genitals. And there is no erotic arousal.

However it is still always my goal to make TPM comfortable and pleasant.

And the practitioner may also add some treatment of the pelvic floor muscles and other pelvic structures, similar to some types of physical therapy. There can even be some mini-chiropractic work on the tail bone part of the spine, from the inside of the pelvis, that some men find beneficial.

If you think that TPM might be useful for you, you might want to investigate the possibility of receiving Therapeutic Prostatic Massage. There is more information on the website.

Epilogue

Thank you for reading Sexy Prostate! And thank you for being willing to take care of your prostate to keep it healthy, problem-free, and ready for pleasure!

If you are interested in medical care for any prostate symptoms or in medical therapeutic prostatic massage, please feel free to contact me via my websites DrErikaMD.com or SexyProstate.com. The previous chapter, Therapeutic Prostatic Massage, gives information about the completely non-sexual nature of this medical modality.

If you have any problems, however minor or major, that are related to prostate problems such as urinary and / or sexual function, please do not continue to suffer: there are ways for you to feel better. So do take action now so that you can enjoy life to the fullest! Don't believe the myth that these issues automatically come with aging and that there is nothing you can do about them. Find the care that you need. Fight the good fight for yourself so that you can be at the top of your game and feel that you have your life back!

Important note: My practice does not include any prostate cancer care. For those problems please contact your urologist or read the websites that you get at the top of the list from an online search. My medical practice only covers prostate problems that are not related to cancer.

Here we are. We've gone through a lot of material in this course. I hope you've learned about the pleasures of prostate massage, as well as ways to deal with the potholes. About all the various places to massage 'down there' and about supplies and positions. Now there is nothing to it but to do it. Do whatever you both can manage. Do it gently and pay attention, and I just bet you'll both be delighted. The biggest prizes go to those who are willing to experiment!

Erika Thost MD
Copyright 2016

Made in the USA
Middletown, DE
11 May 2018